WHAT TURNS YOU ON MORE?

The Sexy Quiz Book for Couples

By

S.W. Taylor

1

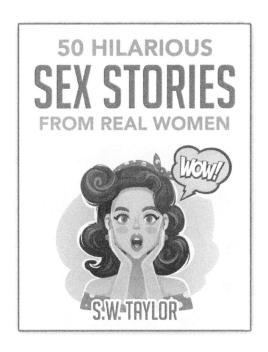

FREE BONUS

READ FOR FREE AT:

SWTBOOKS.COM/FREE

1

WHAT WOULD TURN YOU ON MORE?

Sex with the lights on,

OR

Sex with the lights off?

2

WHAT WOULD TURN YOU ON MORE?

Taking off your partner's underwear with your hands,

OR

Taking off your partner's underwear with your teeth?

3

WHAT WOULD TURN YOU ON MORE?

Having your partner take off your underwear with their hands,

OR

Having your partner pull off your underwear with their teeth?

4

WHAT WOULD TURN YOU ON MORE?

Foreplay with edible underwear,

OR

Foreplay with regular underwear?

5

WHAT WOULD TURN YOU ON MORE?

Giving your partner an oily massage,

OR

Getting an oily massage from your partner?

6

WHAT WOULD TURN YOU ON MORE?

Seeing your partner dressed in a seductive costume,

OR

Seeing your partner completely naked?

7

WHAT WOULD TURN YOU ON MORE?

Getting seduced by a person who doesn't speak your language,

OR

Getting seduced by someone who does?

8

WHAT WOULD TURN YOU ON MORE?

Using a vibrator on your partner,

OR

Having your partner use a vibrator on you?

9

WHAT WOULD TURN
YOU ON MORE?

Being flirted with in the presence of your friends at a club,

OR

Being flirted with while you're alone at a bar?

10

WHAT WOULD TURN
YOU ON MORE?

Watching two people pleasure each other,

OR

Having someone watch while you pleasure your partner?

11

WHAT WOULD TURN YOU ON MORE?

Watching a gay couple have sex,

OR

Watching a straight couple have sex?

12

WHAT WOULD TURN YOU ON MORE?

Being in an open relationship where you and your partner are free to sleep with other people,

OR

Being in an exclusive relationship?

13

WHAT WOULD TURN
YOU ON MORE?

Submitting to your partner's fetish,

OR

Practicing your sexual fetishes on your partner?

14

WHAT WOULD TURN
YOU ON MORE?

Playing your partner's favorite character in bed,

OR

Watching your partner play your favorite character in bed?

15

WHAT WOULD TURN YOU ON MORE?

Visiting a sex club,

OR

Visiting a strip club?

16

WHAT WOULD TURN YOU ON MORE?

Getting thirst traps from your significant other,

OR

Getting thirst traps from a stranger?

17

WHAT WOULD TURN YOU ON MORE?

Receiving nudes from a stranger,

OR

Receiving nudes from your significant other?

18

WHAT WOULD TURN YOU ON MORE?

Getting spanked by your partner randomly,

OR

Spanking your partner when they bend over?

<u>19</u>

WHAT WOULD TURN YOU ON MORE?

Bending your partner over during sex,

OR

Getting bent over by your partner during sex?

<u>20</u>

WHAT WOULD TURN YOU ON MORE?

Getting a hand job under the table in a restaurant,

OR

Getting a hand job in your car?

<u>21</u>

WHAT WOULD TURN YOU ON MORE?

Dirty talk during sex,

OR

Dirty talk before sex?

<u>22</u>

WHAT WOULD TURN YOU ON MORE?

Having a threesome – you and two people of the same gender,

OR

Having a threesome – you and two people of different genders?

23

WHAT WOULD TURN YOU ON MORE?

Bringing someone's sexual fantasies to life,

OR

Having your partner bring your sexual fantasies to life?

24

WHAT WOULD TURN YOU ON MORE?

Having sex with a freaky partner who's open to trying anything,

OR

Having regular but amazing sex?

<u>25</u>

WHAT WOULD TURN YOU ON MORE?

Watching porn videos,

OR

Watching a movie with erotic scenes?

<u>26</u>

WHAT WOULD TURN YOU ON MORE?

Seeing a person scantily clad,

OR

Seeing a person fully clad but with strong sexual appeal?

27

WHAT WOULD TURN
YOU ON MORE?

Having sex with your underwear on,

OR

Having sex completely naked?

28

WHAT WOULD TURN
YOU ON MORE?

Chasing after someone you want in your bed,

OR

Being chased by someone who wants you in their bed?

<u>29</u>

WHAT WOULD TURN YOU ON MORE?

Blindfolding your partner during sex,

OR

Getting blindfolded by your partner during sex?

<u>30</u>

WHAT WOULD TURN YOU ON MORE?

Writing about your best sexual experience,

OR

Reading erotic books?

_30_

WHAT WOULD TURN YOU ON MORE?

Using butt plugs during sex,

OR

Using nipple clamps?

_31_

WHAT WOULD TURN YOU ON MORE?

Playing sexual video games,

OR

Reading erotic magazines?

32

WHAT WOULD TURN YOU ON MORE?

Masturbating with a risk of getting caught,

OR

Masturbating in a locked, comfortable room?

33

WHAT WOULD TURN YOU ON MORE?

Pleasuring yourself,

OR

Getting pleasured by someone else?

34

WHAT WOULD TURN
YOU ON MORE?

Dry humping with your partner while clothed,

OR

Dry humping with your partner while naked?

35

WHAT WOULD TURN
YOU ON MORE?

Seeing your partner half naked,

OR

Seeing your partner completely naked?

<u>36</u>

WHAT WOULD TURN
YOU ON MORE?

Having sex on the kitchen counter,

OR

Having sex on the balcony?

<u>36</u>

WHAT WOULD TURN
YOU ON MORE?

Undressing your partner,

OR

Watching your partner give you a striptease?

37

WHAT WOULD TURN
YOU ON MORE?

Sneakily watching a couple have sex,

OR

Watching a couple have sex with their permission?

38

WHAT WOULD TURN
YOU ON MORE?

Having a threesome,

OR

Having an orgy?

39

WHAT WOULD TURN YOU ON MORE?

Having a threesome with skilled friends,

OR

Having a threesome with experienced strangers?

40

WHAT WOULD TURN YOU ON MORE?

Watching and telling your partner how to touch themselves,

OR

Touching yourself however your partner desires?

<u>41</u>

WHAT WOULD TURN
YOU ON MORE?

Gagging your partner during sex,

OR

Listening to your partner's moans during sex?

<u>42</u>

WHAT WOULD TURN
YOU ON MORE?

Spontaneous sex,

OR

Planned and anticipated sex?

43

WHAT WOULD TURN
YOU ON MORE?

Being seduced by a novice,

OR

Being seduced by a person with experience?

44

WHAT WOULD TURN
YOU ON MORE?

Being creative and making up sexual activities with
a willing partner,

OR

Sticking to regular but mind-blowing sexual
activities?

<u>45</u>

WHAT WOULD TURN YOU ON MORE?

Having sex at a sex club with other couples,

OR

Having sex at home?

<u>45</u>

WHAT WOULD TURN YOU ON MORE?

A quickie in a public place,

OR

Drawn-out sex in a private place?

<u>46</u>

WHAT WOULD TURN YOU ON MORE?

Sex with someone much older than you,

OR

Sex with someone younger than you?

<u>47</u>

WHAT WOULD TURN YOU ON MORE?

Kissing while having sex,

OR

Having sex without kissing?

<u>48</u>

WHAT WOULD TURN YOU ON MORE?

Having sex with a stripper,

OR

Having sex with an acrobat?

<u>49</u>

WHAT WOULD TURN YOU ON MORE?

A person who is rough and experimental in bed,

OR

A person who is gentle and thorough in bed?

50

WHAT WOULD TURN YOU ON MORE?

Flirting with your boss,

OR

Flirting with your co-worker?

51

WHAT WOULD TURN YOU ON MORE?

Having your partner lick wine off your body,

OR

Having your partner eat fruits off your body?

<u>52</u>

WHAT WOULD TURN YOU ON MORE?

Having sex on the first date,

OR

Waiting days to have sex?

<u>53</u>

WHAT WOULD TURN YOU ON MORE?

Sucking on your partner's nipples,

OR

Having your nipples sucked on?

<u>54</u>

WHAT WOULD TURN
YOU ON MORE?

Getting a foot massage,

OR

A back rub?

<u>55</u>

WHAT WOULD TURN
YOU ON MORE?

Being bathed by your partner,

OR

Bathing your partner?

56

WHAT WOULD TURN YOU ON MORE?

Giving your partner head,

OR

Receiving head from your partner?

57

WHAT WOULD TURN YOU ON MORE?

Giving your partner an oily hand job,

OR

Getting a hand job from your partner?

58

WHAT WOULD TURN YOU ON MORE?

Licking whipped cream off your partner's genitals,

OR

Having whipped cream licked off your genitals?

59

WHAT WOULD TURN YOU ON MORE?

Playing with cold temperatures like ice cubes in bed,

OR

Playing with hot temperatures like wax in bed?

60

WHAT WOULD TURN
YOU ON MORE?

Engaging in sexual activities with a person who knows exactly what they want in bed,

OR

Engaging in sexual activities with a flexible person who's willing to try new things?

61

WHAT WOULD TURN
YOU ON MORE?

Hearing your partner commend your skills during sex,

OR

Getting compliments after sex?

<u>62</u>

WHAT WOULD TURN
YOU ON MORE?

Watching your partner do yoga,

OR

Watching your partner dance seductively?

<u>63</u>

WHAT WOULD TURN
YOU ON MORE?

Getting a full-body massage from your partner,

OR

Giving your partner a full-body massage?

<u>64</u>

WHAT WOULD TURN YOU ON MORE?

Hands-off foreplay with only lips and tongues involved,

OR

Foreplay with all parts of the body involved?

<u>65</u>

WHAT WOULD TURN YOU ON MORE?

Having sex against a wall,

OR

Having sex on a chair?

66

WHAT WOULD TURN
YOU ON MORE?

Doing a sixty-nine with your partner,

OR

Doing a seventy-seven with your partner?

67

WHAT WOULD TURN
YOU ON MORE?

Licking your partner's body from head to toe,

OR

Having your partner lick your body from head to toe?

<u>68</u>

WHAT WOULD TURN
YOU ON MORE?

Sex with a little bit of pain involved,

OR

Sex with no pain involved?

<u>69</u>

WHAT WOULD TURN
YOU ON MORE?

Public displays of affection,

OR

Sneaky displays of affection?

<u>70</u>

WHAT WOULD TURN YOU ON MORE?

Getting drunk on wine,

OR

Getting drunk on beer?

<u>71</u>

WHAT WOULD TURN YOU ON MORE?

Watching porn with headphones in public,

OR

Watching porn with the volume up in your room?

<u>72</u>

WHAT WOULD TURN
YOU ON MORE?

Submitting to your partner during sex,

OR

Having a submissive sexual partner?

<u>73</u>

WHAT WOULD TURN
YOU ON MORE?

Having a partner who talks and laughs freely in bed,

OR

Having a partner who concentrates solely on sexual pleasures in bed?

<u>74</u>

WHAT WOULD TURN
YOU ON MORE?

Getting head from someone of the same sex,

OR

Giving head to someone of the same sex?

<u>75</u>

WHAT WOULD TURN
YOU ON MORE?

Watching a girl twerk at a club,

OR

Watching a stripper dance at a club?

<u>76</u>

WHAT WOULD TURN
YOU ON MORE?

Getting a sexy lap dance from a stranger,

OR

Getting a sexy lap dance from your partner?

<u>77</u>

WHAT WOULD TURN
YOU ON MORE?

Having sex with a vocal partner,

OR

Having sex with a non-vocal partner?

<u>78</u>

WHAT WOULD TURN YOU ON MORE?

Doing foreplay outdoors,

OR

Doing foreplay indoors?

<u>79</u>

WHAT WOULD TURN YOU ON MORE?

A slim partner who exercises frequently,

OR

A chubby partner with cute love handles?

80

WHAT WOULD TURN
YOU ON MORE?

A partner with freshly shaved/waxed genitals

OR

A partner with unshaved genitals?

81

WHAT WOULD TURN
YOU ON MORE?

Spontaneous sex after a serious fight,

OR

Sex while laughing and playing with your partner?

82

WHAT WOULD TURN YOU ON MORE?

Anal sex,

OR

Vaginal sex?

83

WHAT WOULD TURN YOU ON MORE?

Playing kinky games with your partner before sex,

OR

No games, sex only?

84

WHAT WOULD TURN YOU ON MORE?

Making a sex tape with your partner,

OR

Making a sex tape with a stranger?

85

WHAT WOULD TURN YOU ON MORE?

Having your partner ride your face,

OR

Giving your partner head while they are lying on their back?

_86_

WHAT WOULD TURN YOU ON MORE?

A strictly sexual relationship,

OR

A committed relationship?

_87_

WHAT WOULD TURN YOU ON MORE?

A sexual partner with tattoos,

OR

A sexual partner without tattoos?

<u>88</u>

WHAT WOULD TURN YOU ON MORE?

A sexual partner with tongue piercings,

OR

A partner with nipple piercings?

<u>89</u>

WHAT WOULD TURN YOU ON MORE?

Dry humping with your partner,

OR

Getting sloppy head from your partner?

<u>90</u>

WHAT WOULD TURN YOU ON MORE?

Getting a hand job in an airplane,

OR

Getting head while driving a car?

<u>91</u>

WHAT WOULD TURN YOU ON MORE?

Phone sex with your partner,

OR

Phone sex with a stranger?

92

WHAT WOULD TURN YOU ON MORE?

Eating fruits off your partner's naked body,

OR

Having your partner eat fruits off your body?

93

WHAT WOULD TURN YOU ON MORE?

A partner who looks innocent but is absolutely freaky in bed,

OR

A partner who is obviously freaky in bed?

94

WHAT WOULD TURN
YOU ON MORE?

Watching your partner play with your genitals,

OR

Playing with your partner's genitals while they watch?

95

WHAT WOULD TURN
YOU ON MORE?

The cowgirl position during sex,

OR

The reverse cowgirl during sex?

<u>96</u>

WHAT WOULD TURN
YOU ON MORE?

Getting a hickey,

OR

Giving your partner a hickey?

<u>97</u>

WHAT WOULD TURN
YOU ON MORE?

Watching someone you are sexually attracted to lick their lips,

OR

Watching them drink from a straw?

98

WHAT WOULD TURN YOU ON MORE?

Sexting with your partner,

OR

Getting nudes from your partner?

99

WHAT WOULD TURN YOU ON MORE?

Watching porn online,

OR

Watching a sex tape of you and your partner?

_100_

WHAT WOULD TURN YOU ON MORE?

Watching straight porn with two people,

OR

Watching a gay threesome?

_101_

WHAT WOULD TURN YOU ON MORE?

Lengthy minutes of thorough foreplay,

OR

Brief seconds of foreplay before getting right to it?

_102_

WHAT WOULD TURN YOU ON MORE?

Seeing your partner approach you completely naked,

OR

Seeing your partner wearing something sexy?

_103_

WHAT WOULD TURN YOU ON MORE?

Dirty talk before sex,

OR

Zero words, actions only?

104

WHAT WOULD TURN YOU ON MORE?

Watching an erotic movie before sex,

OR

Watching an erotic movie during sex?

105

WHAT WOULD TURN YOU ON MORE?

Being dominant in the bedroom,

OR

Being submissive and letting your partner take control?

<u>*106*</u>

WHAT WOULD TURN
YOU ON MORE?

Trying new positions in bed,

OR

Sticking to the sex positions that you already like?

<u>*107*</u>

WHAT WOULD TURN
YOU ON MORE?

Your partner showing you what they like in bed,

OR

Your partner telling you what they like?

_108_

WHAT WOULD TURN YOU ON MORE?

Nude photos,

OR

Steamy lingerie photos for your eyes only?

_109_

WHAT WOULD TURN YOU ON MORE?

A game of truth or dare,

OR

No games, just straight to the bedroom?

110

WHAT WOULD TURN YOU ON MORE?

Sex in a new and unusual place,

OR

Sex in bed?

111

WHAT WOULD TURN YOU ON MORE?

Using sex toys,

OR

No sex toys?

<u>112</u>

WHAT WOULD TURN YOU ON MORE?

Dirty texting,

OR

Dirty talk?

<u>113</u>

WHAT WOULD TURN YOU ON MORE?

A kinky game of truth or dare,

OR

A game of spin the bottle?

<u>114</u>

WHAT WOULD TURN YOU ON MORE?

Your partner in edible underwear,

OR

Your partner in regular underwear?

<u>115</u>

WHAT WOULD TURN YOU ON MORE?

Receiving head from your partner while driving,

OR

Getting a hand job from your partner while driving?

<u>116</u>

WHAT WOULD TURN
YOU ON MORE?

Getting a blow job from your lover,

OR

Giving your lover a blow job?

<u>117</u>

WHAT WOULD TURN
YOU ON MORE?

Watching your partner pleasure themselves,

OR

Pleasuring yourself in front of your partner?

_118_

WHAT WOULD TURN
YOU ON MORE?

Watching your partner make breakfast in nothing
but an apron,

OR

Watching your partner make breakfast in
underwear?

_119_

WHAT WOULD TURN
YOU ON MORE?

Rough sex,

OR

Slow, sensual lovemaking?

<u>120</u>

WHAT WOULD TURN
YOU ON MORE?

Oral sex in the car,

OR

A hand job under the dinner table?

<u>121</u>

WHAT WOULD TURN
YOU ON MORE?

A bold, direct invitation to the bedroom,

OR

A subtle, hinted at invitation to the bedroom?

_122_

WHAT WOULD TURN
YOU ON MORE?

Sex with more than one person –a threesome,

OR

Sex with one partner?

_123_

WHAT WOULD TURN
YOU ON MORE?

Being bound to the bed,

OR

Having sex unbound?

<u>124</u>

WHAT WOULD TURN
YOU ON MORE?

Being choked by your partner during sex,

OR

Being spanked?

<u>125</u>

WHAT WOULD TURN
YOU ON MORE?

Licking chocolate off your partner's body,

OR

Having chocolate eaten off your body?

126

WHAT WOULD TURN YOU ON MORE?

Getting a lap dance at a club,

OR

Giving a lap dance at a club?

127

WHAT WOULD TURN YOU ON MORE?

Getting sexually intimate in a public place, like a cinema,

OR

Getting sexually intimate in a private place like your bedroom or a hotel room?

_128_

WHAT WOULD TURN
YOU ON MORE?

A long French kiss,

OR

Kisses on the neck?

_129_

WHAT WOULD TURN
YOU ON MORE?

A foot massage,

OR

A back massage?

130

WHAT WOULD TURN
YOU ON MORE?

Taking a shower with your partner,

OR

Skinny-dipping with your partner?

131

WHAT WOULD TURN
YOU ON MORE?

A sensual playlist on the radio,

OR

A steamy movie on the television?

<u>132</u>

WHAT WOULD TURN
YOU ON MORE?

Watching strippers at a club,

OR

Getting a private striptease in your bedroom?

<u>133</u>

WHAT WOULD TURN
YOU ON MORE?

Watching gay porn,

OR

Watching heterosexual porn?

134

WHAT WOULD TURN YOU ON MORE?

BDSM with your partner,

OR

Gentle lovemaking?

135

WHAT WOULD TURN YOU ON MORE?

Having sex while lying on a bed,

OR

Having sex bent over on a balcony?

<u>136</u>

WHAT WOULD TURN YOU ON MORE?

Being seduced by someone,

OR

Seducing someone?

<u>137</u>

WHAT WOULD TURN YOU ON MORE?

Talking about previous sexual experiences,

OR

Sharing your sexual fantasies?

138

WHAT WOULD TURN
YOU ON MORE?

Dirty texting in public,

OR

Dirty texting in private?

139

WHAT WOULD TURN
YOU ON MORE?

Touching yourself in private,

OR

Touching yourself in the presence of someone else?

140

WHAT WOULD TURN YOU ON MORE?

Using sexual toys on yourself,

OR

Using sexual toys on your partner?

141

WHAT WOULD TURN YOU ON MORE?

The thought of a quickie in a dressing room,

OR

Lengthy sex in a bedroom?

<u>142</u>

WHAT WOULD TURN
YOU ON MORE?

A one-night stand with a stranger you may never see again,

OR

A one night stand with a friend?

<u>143</u>

WHAT WOULD TURN
YOU ON MORE?

Being blindfolded during foreplay and sex,

OR

Being handcuffed during foreplay and sex?

144

WHAT WOULD TURN
YOU ON MORE?

Watching a couple have sex with their permission,

OR

Being watched by a couple while you have sex?

145

WHAT WOULD TURN
YOU ON MORE?

Dry humping with your partner,

OR

Receiving a hand job from your partner?

146

WHAT WOULD TURN YOU ON MORE?

Drinking wine off your partner's body,

OR

Having your partner drink wine off your body?

147

WHAT WOULD TURN YOU ON MORE?

Using ice in the bedroom,

OR

Using wax in the bedroom?

<u>148</u>

WHAT WOULD TURN
YOU ON MORE?

A partner that moans/groans loudly,

OR

A quiet partner?

<u>149</u>

WHAT WOULD TURN
YOU ON MORE?

Biting your partner,

OR

Getting bitten by your partner?

150

WHAT WOULD TURN YOU ON MORE?

Dirty dancing with someone in a club,

OR

Dirty dancing with your partner in the living room?

151

WHAT WOULD TURN YOU ON MORE?

Teasing your partner during foreplay,

OR

Getting teased by your partner during foreplay?

<u>152</u>

WHAT WOULD TURN
YOU ON MORE?

Kissing a person of the opposite sex,

OR

Kissing someone of the same sex?

<u>153</u>

WHAT WOULD TURN
YOU ON MORE?

Watching your partner take a shower,

OR

Taking a shower with your partner?

154

WHAT WOULD TURN YOU ON MORE?

Receiving a naughty picture,

OR

Sending a naughty picture?

155

WHAT WOULD TURN YOU ON MORE?

Seeing your partner in pants only,

OR

Seeing your partner in a shirt or blouse only?

156

WHAT WOULD TURN
YOU ON MORE?

Tying up your partner in the bedroom,

OR

Being tied up by your partner in the bedroom?

157

WHAT WOULD TURN
YOU ON MORE?

Sex in the back of the car,

OR

Sex in the front seat?

158

WHAT WOULD TURN
YOU ON MORE?

Watching your partner reach orgasm,

OR

Reaching orgasm while your partner watches?

159

WHAT WOULD TURN
YOU ON MORE?

Getting videos of your partner playing with themselves,

OR

Getting pictures of your partner in lingerie?

_160_

WHAT WOULD TURN
YOU ON MORE?

A sexual relationship with a random friend,

OR

A sexual relationship with a committed partner?

_161_

WHAT WOULD TURN
YOU ON MORE?

Your partner wearing nothing but stilettoes,

OR

Your partner wearing nothing at all?

162

WHAT WOULD TURN YOU ON MORE?

Listening to dirty talk,

OR

You talking dirty to your partner?

163

WHAT WOULD TURN YOU ON MORE?

Making the first move on your partner,

OR

Having your partner make the first move to seduce you?

<u>164</u>

WHAT WOULD TURN
YOU ON MORE?

A room lit with candles and covered in roses,

OR

A well-lit room where you can see your partner clearly?

<u>165</u>

WHAT WOULD TURN
YOU ON MORE?

Having your hair pulled during sex,

OR

Pulling your partner's hair during sex?

_166_

WHAT WOULD TURN YOU ON MORE?

Having sex missionary style,

OR

Having sex doggy style?

_167_

WHAT WOULD TURN YOU ON MORE?

Lying on your back during sex,

OR

Being on top during sex?

168

WHAT WOULD TURN YOU ON MORE?

Sexual activities with a person you love,

OR

Sexual activities with a stranger?

169

WHAT WOULD TURN YOU ON MORE?

Eating off your partner's naked body,

OR

Drinking off your partner's naked body?

170

WHAT WOULD TURN YOU ON MORE?

A big butt and small breasts,

OR

A small butt and big breasts?

171

WHAT WOULD TURN YOU ON MORE?

Foreplay in a movie theater with the risk of being seen by passersby,

OR

Foreplay in a place where no one can see you?

<u>172</u>

WHAT WOULD TURN YOU ON MORE?

Having sex in the daytime,

OR

Having sex at night?

<u>173</u>

WHAT WOULD TURN YOU ON MORE?

Seeing your partner dress up as an angel,

OR

Seeing your partner dress up as a demon?

<u>174</u>

WHAT WOULD TURN
YOU ON MORE?

Sex with protection,

OR

Sex without protection?

<u>175</u>

WHAT WOULD TURN
YOU ON MORE?

Chasing after someone who plays hard to get,

OR

No chase, just straight to the bedroom?

<u>176</u>

WHAT WOULD TURN
YOU ON MORE?

Being in an open relationship,

OR

Being in an exclusive relationship?

<u>177</u>

WHAT WOULD TURN
YOU ON MORE?

Watching your partner win an argument,

OR

Watching your partner smile?

178

WHAT WOULD TURN YOU ON MORE?

Having sex in a place you shouldn't be caught having sex,

OR

Having sex in a comfortable and appropriate setting?

179

WHAT WOULD TURN YOU ON MORE?

Having sex with someone you should not be having sex with,

OR

Having sex with your partner?

180

WHAT WOULD TURN
YOU ON MORE?

Getting sexually intimate with your partner with the lights on,

OR

Getting sexually intimate with your partner with the lights off?

181

WHAT WOULD TURN
YOU ON MORE?

Having amazing missionary-style sex with your partner,

OR

Trying different, exciting new sexual positions with your partner?

<u>182</u>

WHAT WOULD TURN
YOU ON MORE?

Having sexual dreams,

OR

Having sexual fantasies?

<u>183</u>

WHAT WOULD TURN
YOU ON MORE?

Sex with someone inexperienced but willing to learn new things,

OR

Sex with an experienced person?

184

WHAT WOULD TURN
YOU ON MORE?

Experiencing slight, exciting pain during sex,

OR

Sex without any pain?

185

WHAT WOULD TURN
YOU ON MORE?

A partner who can have numerous rounds of sex,

OR

A partner who will make one round of sex mind-blowing?

186

WHAT WOULD TURN YOU ON MORE?

Sex with a person from a different race,

OR

Sex with someone from your race?

187

WHAT WOULD TURN YOU ON MORE?

Watching a movie sex scene alone,

OR

Watching a movie sex scene with a group of people?

188

WHAT WOULD TURN YOU ON MORE?

Reading an erotic book,

OR

Watching an erotic movie?

189

WHAT WOULD TURN YOU ON MORE?

Having stimulating voice phone sex,

OR

Having exciting video phone sex?

190

WHAT WOULD TURN
YOU ON MORE?

Watching your partner slowly lick candy,

OR

Watching your partner slowly eat a banana?

191

WHAT WOULD TURN
YOU ON MORE?

Watching a threesome porn video,

OR

Watching an orgy?

<u>192</u>

WHAT WOULD TURN YOU ON MORE?

Dirty talk over the phone,

OR

Naked Facetime?

<u>193</u>

WHAT WOULD TURN YOU ON MORE?

A flexible partner who can be acrobatic in bed,

OR

A non-acrobatic partner who knows all the places you like to be touched?

<u>194</u>

WHAT WOULD TURN
YOU ON MORE?

Listening to erotic music while touching yourself,

OR

Watching porn while touching yourself?

<u>195</u>

WHAT WOULD TURN
YOU ON MORE?

Having sex on a bed,

OR

Having sex on a couch?

<u>196</u>

WHAT WOULD TURN YOU ON MORE?

Touching yourself,

OR

Having someone touch you?

<u>197</u>

WHAT WOULD TURN YOU ON MORE?

Having sex completely naked,

OR

Having sex half clothed?

198

WHAT WOULD TURN
YOU ON MORE?

Using sex toys on your partner,

OR

Having your partner use sex toys on you?

199

WHAT WOULD TURN
YOU ON MORE?

Trying different positions during sex,

OR

Sticking to one (the best) position during sex?

200

WHAT WOULD TURN YOU ON MORE?

Sneaking around with the person you're having sex with,

OR

Being bold and direct about your sexual relationship with that person?

Final Words

We hope you enjoyed the book!

Please consider leaving a review by going to:

SWTBOOKS.COM/REVIEW

40147851R00066